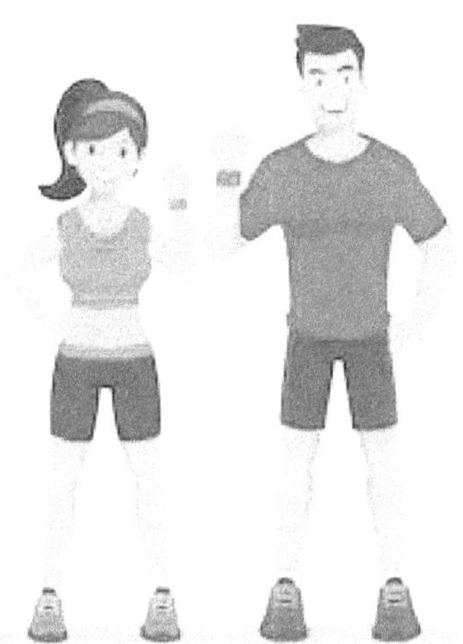

Fitness Day After Day

After Waking up

Write your weight after wakeup

My Weight is	

In The Gym

Write the hours you spent in the gym

Gym Hours	

Before Sleeping

Write your weight before go to bed

My Weight is	

Lose weight

Subtract the 2 weights to know
how many grams you lose

I lose	Grams

After Waking up

Write your weight after wakeup

My Weight is	

In The Gym

Write the hours you spent in the gym

Gym Hours	

Before Sleeping

Write your weight before go to bed

My Weight is	

Lose weight

Subtract the 2 weights to know
how many grams you lose

I lose	Grams

After Waking up

Write your weight after wakeup

My Weight is	

In The Gym

Write the hours you spent in the gym

Gym Hours	

Before Sleeping

Write your weight before go to bed

My Weight is	

Lose weight

Subtract the 2 weights to know
how many grams you lose

I lose		Grams

After Waking up

Write your weight after wakeup

My Weight is	

In The Gym

Write the hours you spent in the gym

Gym Hours	

Before Sleeping

Write your weight before go to bed

My Weight is	

Lose weight

Subtract the 2 weights to know
how many grams you lose

I lose	Grams

After Waking up

Write your weight after wakeup

My Weight is	

In The Gym

Write the hours you spent in the gym

Gym Hours	

Before Sleeping

Write your weight before go to bed

My Weight is	

Lose weight

Subtract the 2 weights to know
how many grams you lose

I lose	Grams

After Waking up

Write your weight after wakeup

My Weight is	

In The Gym

Write the hours you spent in the gym

Gym Hours	

Before Sleeping

Write your weight before go to bed

My Weight is	

Lose weight

Subtract the 2 weights to know
how many grams you lose

I lose	Grams

After Waking up

Write your weight after wakeup

My Weight is	

In The Gym

Write the hours you spent in the gym

Gym Hours	

Before Sleeping

Write your weight before go to bed

My Weight is	

Lose weight

Subtract the 2 weights to know
how many grams you lose

I lose		Grams

After Waking up

Write your weight after wakeup

My Weight is	

In The Gym

Write the hours you spent in the gym

Gym Hours	

Before Sleeping

Write your weight before go to bed

My Weight is	

Lose weight

Subtract the 2 weights to know
how many grams you lose

I lose	Grams

After Waking up

Write your weight after wakeup

My Weight is	

In The Gym

Write the hours you spent in the gym

Gym Hours	

Before Sleeping

Write your weight before go to bed

My Weight is	

Lose weight

Subtract the 2 weights to know
how many grams you lose

I lose		Grams

After Waking up

Write your weight after wakeup

My Weight is	

In The Gym

Write the hours you spent in the gym

Gym Hours	

Before Sleeping

Write your weight before go to bed

My Weight is	

Lose weight

Subtract the 2 weights to know
how many grams you lose

I lose	Grams

After Waking up

Write your weight after wakeup

My Weight is	

In The Gym

Write the hours you spent in the gym

Gym Hours	

Before Sleeping

Write your weight before go to bed

My Weight is	

Lose weight

Subtract the 2 weights to know
how many grams you lose

I lose		Grams

After Waking up

Write your weight after wakeup

My Weight is	

In The Gym

Write the hours you spent in the gym

Gym Hours	

Before Sleeping

Write your weight before go to bed

My Weight is	

Lose weight

Subtract the 2 weights to know
how many grams you lose

I lose	Grams

After Waking up

Write your weight after wakeup

My Weight is	

In The Gym

Write the hours you spent in the gym

Gym Hours	

Before Sleeping

Write your weight before go to bed

My Weight is	

Lose weight

Subtract the 2 weights to know
how many grams you lose

I lose	Grams

After Waking up

Write your weight after wakeup

My Weight is	

In The Gym

Write the hours you spent in the gym

Gym Hours	

Before Sleeping

Write your weight before go to bed

My Weight is	

Lose weight

Subtract the 2 weights to know
how many grams you lose

I lose	Grams

After Waking up

Write your weight after wakeup

My Weight is	

In The Gym

Write the hours you spent in the gym

Gym Hours	

Before Sleeping

Write your weight before go to bed

My Weight is	

Lose weight

Subtract the 2 weights to know
how many grams you lose

I lose	Grams

After Waking up

Write your weight after wakeup

My Weight is	

In The Gym

Write the hours you spent in the gym

Gym Hours	

Before Sleeping

Write your weight before go to bed

My Weight is	

Lose weight

Subtract the 2 weights to know
how many grams you lose

I lose	Grams

After Waking up

Write your weight after wakeup

My Weight is	

In The Gym

Write the hours you spent in the gym

Gym Hours	

Before Sleeping

Write your weight before go to bed

My Weight is	

Lose weight

Subtract the 2 weights to know
how many grams you lose

I lose	Grams

After Waking up

Write your weight after wakeup

My Weight is	

In The Gym

Write the hours you spent in the gym

Gym Hours	

Before Sleeping

Write your weight before go to bed

My Weight is	

Lose weight

Subtract the 2 weights to know
how many grams you lose

I lose	Grams

After Waking up

Write your weight after wakeup

My Weight is	

In The Gym

Write the hours you spent in the gym

Gym Hours	

Before Sleeping

Write your weight before go to bed

My Weight is	

Lose weight

Subtract the 2 weights to know
how many grams you lose

I lose		Grams

After Waking up

Write your weight after wakeup

My Weight is	

In The Gym

Write the hours you spent in the gym

Gym Hours	

Before Sleeping

Write your weight before go to bed

My Weight is	

Lose weight

Subtract the 2 weights to know
how many grams you lose

I lose	Grams

After Waking up

Write your weight after wakeup

My Weight is	

In The Gym

Write the hours you spent in the gym

Gym Hours	

Before Sleeping

Write your weight before go to bed

My Weight is	

Lose weight

Subtract the 2 weights to know
how many grams you lose

I lose		Grams

After Waking up

Write your weight after wakeup

My Weight is	

In The Gym

Write the hours you spent in the gym

Gym Hours	

Before Sleeping

Write your weight before go to bed

My Weight is	

Lose weight

Subtract the 2 weights to know
how many grams you lose

I lose	Grams

After Waking up

Write your weight after wakeup

My Weight is	

In The Gym

Write the hours you spent in the gym

Gym Hours	

Before Sleeping

Write your weight before go to bed

My Weight is	

Lose weight

Subtract the 2 weights to know
how many grams you lose

I lose	Grams

After Waking up

Write your weight after wakeup

My Weight is	

In The Gym

Write the hours you spent in the gym

Gym Hours	

Before Sleeping

Write your weight before go to bed

My Weight is	

Lose weight

Subtract the 2 weights to know
how many grams you lose

I lose	Grams

After Waking up

Write your weight after wakeup

My Weight is	

In The Gym

Write the hours you spent in the gym

Gym Hours	

Before Sleeping

Write your weight before go to bed

My Weight is	

Lose weight

Subtract the 2 weights to know
how many grams you lose

I lose		Grams

After Waking up

Write your weight after wakeup

My Weight is	

In The Gym

Write the hours you spent in the gym

Gym Hours	

Before Sleeping

Write your weight before go to bed

My Weight is	

Lose weight

Subtract the 2 weights to know
how many grams you lose

I lose	Grams

After Waking up

Write your weight after wakeup

My Weight is	

In The Gym

Write the hours you spent in the gym

Gym Hours	

Before Sleeping

Write your weight before go to bed

My Weight is	

Lose weight

Subtract the 2 weights to know
how many grams you lose

I lose	Grams

After Waking up

Write your weight after wakeup

My Weight is	

In The Gym

Write the hours you spent in the gym

Gym Hours	

Before Sleeping

Write your weight before go to bed

My Weight is	

Lose weight

Subtract the 2 weights to know
how many grams you lose

I lose	Grams

After Waking up

Write your weight after wakeup

My Weight is	

In The Gym

Write the hours you spent in the gym

Gym Hours	

Before Sleeping

Write your weight before go to bed

My Weight is	

Lose weight

Subtract the 2 weights to know
how many grams you lose

I lose	Grams

After Waking up

Write your weight after wakeup

My Weight is	

In The Gym

Write the hours you spent in the gym

Gym Hours	

Before Sleeping

Write your weight before go to bed

My Weight is	

Lose weight

Subtract the 2 weights to know
how many grams you lose

I lose	Grams

After Waking up

Write your weight after wakeup

My Weight is	

In The Gym

Write the hours you spent in the gym

Gym Hours	

Before Sleeping

Write your weight before go to bed

My Weight is	

Lose weight

Subtract the 2 weights to know
how many grams you lose

I lose	Grams

After Waking up

Write your weight after wakeup

My Weight is	

In The Gym

Write the hours you spent in the gym

Gym Hours	

Before Sleeping

Write your weight before go to bed

My Weight is	

Lose weight

Subtract the 2 weights to know
how many grams you lose

I lose	Grams

After Waking up

Write your weight after wakeup

My Weight is	

In The Gym

Write the hours you spent in the gym

Gym Hours	

Before Sleeping

Write your weight before go to bed

My Weight is	

Lose weight

Subtract the 2 weights to know
how many grams you lose

I lose	Grams

After Waking up

Write your weight after wakeup

My Weight is	

In The Gym

Write the hours you spent in the gym

Gym Hours	

Before Sleeping

Write your weight before go to bed

My Weight is	

Lose weight

Subtract the 2 weights to know
how many grams you lose

I lose	Grams

After Waking up

Write your weight after wakeup

My Weight is	

In The Gym

Write the hours you spent in the gym

Gym Hours	

Before Sleeping

Write your weight before go to bed

My Weight is	

Lose weight

Subtract the 2 weights to know
how many grams you lose

I lose	Grams

After Waking up

Write your weight after wakeup

My Weight is	

In The Gym

Write the hours you spent in the gym

Gym Hours	

Before Sleeping

Write your weight before go to bed

My Weight is	

Lose weight

Subtract the 2 weights to know
how many grams you lose

I lose	Grams

After Waking up

Write your weight after wakeup

My Weight is	

In The Gym

Write the hours you spent in the gym

Gym Hours	

Before Sleeping

Write your weight before go to bed

My Weight is	

Lose weight

Subtract the 2 weights to know
how many grams you lose

I lose		Grams

After Waking up

Write your weight after wakeup

My Weight is	

In The Gym

Write the hours you spent in the gym

Gym Hours	

Before Sleeping

Write your weight before go to bed

My Weight is	

Lose weight

Subtract the 2 weights to know
how many grams you lose

I lose	Grams

After Waking up

Write your weight after wakeup

My Weight is	

In The Gym

Write the hours you spent in the gym

Gym Hours	

Before Sleeping

Write your weight before go to bed

My Weight is	

Lose weight

Subtract the 2 weights to know
how many grams you lose

I lose		Grams

After Waking up

Write your weight after wakeup

My Weight is	

In The Gym

Write the hours you spent in the gym

Gym Hours	

Before Sleeping

Write your weight before go to bed

My Weight is	

Lose weight

Subtract the 2 weights to know
how many grams you lose

I lose	Grams

After Waking up

Write your weight after wakeup

My Weight is	

In The Gym

Write the hours you spent in the gym

Gym Hours	

Before Sleeping

Write your weight before go to bed

My Weight is	

Lose weight

Subtract the 2 weights to know
how many grams you lose

I lose	Grams

After Waking up

Write your weight after wakeup

My Weight is	

In The Gym

Write the hours you spent in the gym

Gym Hours	

Before Sleeping

Write your weight before go to bed

My Weight is	

Lose weight

Subtract the 2 weights to know
how many grams you lose

I lose	Grams

After Waking up

Write your weight after wakeup

My Weight is	

In The Gym

Write the hours you spent in the gym

Gym Hours	

Before Sleeping

Write your weight before go to bed

My Weight is	

Lose weight

Subtract the 2 weights to know
how many grams you lose

I lose	Grams

Copy righted image

After Waking up

Write your weight after wakeup

My Weight is	

In The Gym

Write the hours you spent in the gym

Gym Hours	

Before Sleeping

Write your weight before go to bed

My Weight is	

Lose weight

Subtract the 2 weights to know
how many grams you lose

I lose	Grams

After Waking up

Write your weight after wakeup

My Weight is	

In The Gym

Write the hours you spent in the gym

Gym Hours	

Before Sleeping

Write your weight before go to bed

My Weight is	

Lose weight

Subtract the 2 weights to know
how many grams you lose

I lose	Grams

After Waking up

Write your weight after wakeup

My Weight is	

In The Gym

Write the hours you spent in the gym

Gym Hours	

Before Sleeping

Write your weight before go to bed

My Weight is	

Lose weight

Subtract the 2 weights to know
how many grams you lose

I lose		Grams

After Waking up

Write your weight after wakeup

My Weight is	

In The Gym

Write the hours you spent in the gym

Gym Hours	

Before Sleeping

Write your weight before go to bed

My Weight is	

Lose weight

Subtract the 2 weights to know
how many grams you lose

I lose	Grams

After Waking up

Write your weight after wakeup

My Weight is	

In The Gym

Write the hours you spent in the gym

Gym Hours	

Before Sleeping

Write your weight before go to bed

My Weight is	

Lose weight

Subtract the 2 weights to know
how many grams you lose

I lose	Grams

After Waking up

Write your weight after wakeup

My Weight is	

In The Gym

Write the hours you spent in the gym

Gym Hours	

Before Sleeping

Write your weight before go to bed

My Weight is	

Lose weight

Subtract the 2 weights to know
how many grams you lose

I lose		Grams

After Waking up

Write your weight after wakeup

My Weight is	

In The Gym

Write the hours you spent in the gym

Gym Hours	

Before Sleeping

Write your weight before go to bed

My Weight is	

Lose weight

Subtract the 2 weights to know
how many grams you lose

I lose	Grams

After Waking up

Write your weight after wakeup

My Weight is	

In The Gym

Write the hours you spent in the gym

Gym Hours	

Before Sleeping

Write your weight before go to bed

My Weight is	

Lose weight

Subtract the 2 weights to know
how many grams you lose

I lose		Grams

After Waking up

Write your weight after wakeup

My Weight is	

In The Gym

Write the hours you spent in the gym

Gym Hours	

Before Sleeping

Write your weight before go to bed

My Weight is	

Lose weight

Subtract the 2 weights to know
how many grams you lose

I lose	Grams

After Waking up

Write your weight after wakeup

My Weight is	

In The Gym

Write the hours you spent in the gym

Gym Hours	

Before Sleeping

Write your weight before go to bed

My Weight is	

Lose weight

Subtract the 2 weights to know
how many grams you lose

I lose	Grams

After Waking up

Write your weight after wakeup

My Weight is	

In The Gym

Write the hours you spent in the gym

Gym Hours	

Before Sleeping

Write your weight before go to bed

My Weight is	

Lose weight

Subtract the 2 weights to know
how many grams you lose

I lose		Grams

After Waking up

Write your weight after wakeup

My Weight is	

In The Gym

Write the hours you spent in the gym

Gym Hours	

Before Sleeping

Write your weight before go to bed

My Weight is	

Lose weight

Subtract the 2 weights to know
how many grams you lose

I lose	Grams

After Waking up

Write your weight after wakeup

My Weight is	

In The Gym

Write the hours you spent in the gym

Gym Hours	

Before Sleeping

Write your weight before go to bed

My Weight is	

Lose weight

Subtract the 2 weights to know
how many grams you lose

I lose	Grams

After Waking up

Write your weight after wakeup

My Weight is	

In The Gym

Write the hours you spent in the gym

Gym Hours	

Before Sleeping

Write your weight before go to bed

My Weight is	

Lose weight

Subtract the 2 weights to know
how many grams you lose

I lose	Grams

After Waking up

Write your weight after wakeup

My Weight is	

In The Gym

Write the hours you spent in the gym

Gym Hours	

Before Sleeping

Write your weight before go to bed

My Weight is	

Lose weight

Subtract the 2 weights to know
how many grams you lose

I lose	Grams

After Waking up

Write your weight after wakeup

My Weight is	

In The Gym

Write the hours you spent in the gym

Gym Hours	

Before Sleeping

Write your weight before go to bed

My Weight is	

Lose weight

Subtract the 2 weights to know
how many grams you lose

I lose	Grams

After Waking up

Write your weight after wakeup

My Weight is	

In The Gym

Write the hours you spent in the gym

Gym Hours	

Before Sleeping

Write your weight before go to bed

My Weight is	

Lose weight

Subtract the 2 weights to know
how many grams you lose

I lose	Grams

After Waking up

Write your weight after wakeup

My Weight is	

In The Gym

Write the hours you spent in the gym

Gym Hours	

Before Sleeping

Write your weight before go to bed

My Weight is	

Lose weight

Subtract the 2 weights to know
how many grams you lose

I lose	Grams

Copy righted image

After Waking up

Write your weight after wakeup

My Weight is	

In The Gym

Write the hours you spent in the gym

Gym Hours	

Before Sleeping

Write your weight before go to bed

My Weight is	

Lose weight

Subtract the 2 weights to know
how many grams you lose

I lose	Grams

After Waking up

Write your weight after wakeup

My Weight is	

In The Gym

Write the hours you spent in the gym

Gym Hours	

Before Sleeping

Write your weight before go to bed

My Weight is	

Lose weight

Subtract the 2 weights to know
how many grams you lose

I lose	Grams

After Waking up

Write your weight after wakeup

My Weight is	

In The Gym

Write the hours you spent in the gym

Gym Hours	

Before Sleeping

Write your weight before go to bed

My Weight is	

Lose weight

Subtract the 2 weights to know
how many grams you lose

I lose	Grams

After Waking up

Write your weight after wakeup

My Weight is	

In The Gym

Write the hours you spent in the gym

Gym Hours	

Before Sleeping

Write your weight before go to bed

My Weight is	

Lose weight

Subtract the 2 weights to know
how many grams you lose

I lose	Grams

After Waking up

Write your weight after wakeup

My Weight is	

In The Gym

Write the hours you spent in the gym

Gym Hours	

Before Sleeping

Write your weight before go to bed

My Weight is	

Lose weight

Subtract the 2 weights to know
how many grams you lose

I lose	Grams

After Waking up

Write your weight after wakeup

My Weight is	

In The Gym

Write the hours you spent in the gym

Gym Hours	

Before Sleeping

Write your weight before go to bed

My Weight is	

Lose weight

Subtract the 2 weights to know
how many grams you lose

I lose		Grams

After Waking up

Write your weight after wakeup

My Weight is	

In The Gym

Write the hours you spent in the gym

Gym Hours	

Before Sleeping

Write your weight before go to bed

My Weight is	

Lose weight

Subtract the 2 weights to know
how many grams you lose

I lose		Grams

After Waking up

Write your weight after wakeup

My Weight is	

In The Gym

Write the hours you spent in the gym

Gym Hours	

Before Sleeping

Write your weight before go to bed

My Weight is	

Lose weight

Subtract the 2 weights to know
how many grams you lose

I lose	Grams

After Waking up

Write your weight after wakeup

My Weight is	

In The Gym

Write the hours you spent in the gym

Gym Hours	

Before Sleeping

Write your weight before go to bed

My Weight is	

Lose weight

Subtract the 2 weights to know
how many grams you lose

I lose	Grams

After Waking up

Write your weight after wakeup

My Weight is	

In The Gym

Write the hours you spent in the gym

Gym Hours	

Before Sleeping

Write your weight before go to bed

My Weight is	

Lose weight

Subtract the 2 weights to know
how many grams you lose

I lose	Grams

After Waking up

Write your weight after wakeup

My Weight is	

In The Gym

Write the hours you spent in the gym

Gym Hours	

Before Sleeping

Write your weight before go to bed

My Weight is	

Lose weight

Subtract the 2 weights to know
how many grams you lose

I lose	Grams

After Waking up

Write your weight after wakeup

My Weight is	

In The Gym

Write the hours you spent in the gym

Gym Hours	

Before Sleeping

Write your weight before go to bed

My Weight is	

Lose weight

Subtract the 2 weights to know
how many grams you lose

I lose		Grams

After Waking up

Write your weight after wakeup

My Weight is	

In The Gym

Write the hours you spent in the gym

Gym Hours	

Before Sleeping

Write your weight before go to bed

My Weight is	

Lose weight

Subtract the 2 weights to know
how many grams you lose

I lose	Grams

After Waking up

Write your weight after wakeup

My Weight is	

In The Gym

Write the hours you spent in the gym

Gym Hours	

Before Sleeping

Write your weight before go to bed

My Weight is	

Lose weight

Subtract the 2 weights to know
how many grams you lose

I lose		Grams

After Waking up

Write your weight after wakeup

My Weight is	

In The Gym

Write the hours you spent in the gym

Gym Hours	

Before Sleeping

Write your weight before go to bed

My Weight is	

Lose weight

Subtract the 2 weights to know
how many grams you lose

I lose	Grams

After Waking up

Write your weight after wakeup

My Weight is	

In The Gym

Write the hours you spent in the gym

Gym Hours	

Before Sleeping

Write your weight before go to bed

My Weight is	

Lose weight

Subtract the 2 weights to know
how many grams you lose

I lose	Grams

After Waking up

Write your weight after wakeup

My Weight is	

In The Gym

Write the hours you spent in the gym

Gym Hours	

Before Sleeping

Write your weight before go to bed

My Weight is	

Lose weight

Subtract the 2 weights to know
how many grams you lose

I lose	Grams

After Waking up

Write your weight after wakeup

My Weight is	

In The Gym

Write the hours you spent in the gym

Gym Hours	

Before Sleeping

Write your weight before go to bed

My Weight is	

Lose weight

Subtract the 2 weights to know
how many grams you lose

I lose	Grams

After Waking up

Write your weight after wakeup

My Weight is	

In The Gym

Write the hours you spent in the gym

Gym Hours	

Before Sleeping

Write your weight before go to bed

My Weight is	

Lose weight

Subtract the 2 weights to know
how many grams you lose

I lose	Grams

After Waking up

Write your weight after wakeup

My Weight is	

In The Gym

Write the hours you spent in the gym

Gym Hours	

Before Sleeping

Write your weight before go to bed

My Weight is	

Lose weight

Subtract the 2 weights to know
how many grams you lose

I lose	Grams

After Waking up

Write your weight after wakeup

My Weight is	

In The Gym

Write the hours you spent in the gym

Gym Hours	

Before Sleeping

Write your weight before go to bed

My Weight is	

Lose weight

Subtract the 2 weights to know
how many grams you lose

I lose	Grams

After Waking up

Write your weight after wakeup

My Weight is	

In The Gym

Write the hours you spent in the gym

Gym Hours	

Before Sleeping

Write your weight before go to bed

My Weight is	

Lose weight

Subtract the 2 weights to know
how many grams you lose

I lose	Grams

After Waking up

Write your weight after wakeup

My Weight is	

In The Gym

Write the hours you spent in the gym

Gym Hours	

Before Sleeping

Write your weight before go to bed

My Weight is	

Lose weight

Subtract the 2 weights to know
how many grams you lose

I lose	Grams

After Waking up

Write your weight after wakeup

My Weight is	

In The Gym

Write the hours you spent in the gym

Gym Hours	

Before Sleeping

Write your weight before go to bed

My Weight is	

Lose weight

Subtract the 2 weights to know
how many grams you lose

I lose	Grams

After Waking up

Write your weight after wakeup

My Weight is	

In The Gym

Write the hours you spent in the gym

Gym Hours	

Before Sleeping

Write your weight before go to bed

My Weight is	

Lose weight

Subtract the 2 weights to know
how many grams you lose

I lose	Grams

After Waking up

Write your weight after wakeup

My Weight is	

In The Gym

Write the hours you spent in the gym

Gym Hours	

Before Sleeping

Write your weight before go to bed

My Weight is	

Lose weight

Subtract the 2 weights to know
how many grams you lose

I lose	Grams

After Waking up

Write your weight after wakeup

My Weight is	

In The Gym

Write the hours you spent in the gym

Gym Hours	

Before Sleeping

Write your weight before go to bed

My Weight is	

Lose weight

Subtract the 2 weights to know
how many grams you lose

I lose	Grams

After Waking up

Write your weight after wakeup

My Weight is	

In The Gym

Write the hours you spent in the gym

Gym Hours	

Before Sleeping

Write your weight before go to bed

My Weight is	

Lose weight

Subtract the 2 weights to know
how many grams you lose

I lose	Grams

After Waking up

Write your weight after wakeup

My Weight is	

In The Gym

Write the hours you spent in the gym

Gym Hours	

Before Sleeping

Write your weight before go to bed

My Weight is	

Lose weight

Subtract the 2 weights to know
how many grams you lose

I lose	Grams

After Waking up

Write your weight after wakeup

My Weight is	

In The Gym

Write the hours you spent in the gym

Gym Hours	

Before Sleeping

Write your weight before go to bed

My Weight is	

Lose weight

Subtract the 2 weights to know
how many grams you lose

I lose		Grams

Copy righted image

After Waking up

Write your weight after wakeup

My Weight is	

In The Gym

Write the hours you spent in the gym

Gym Hours	

Before Sleeping

Write your weight before go to bed

My Weight is	

Lose weight

Subtract the 2 weights to know
how many grams you lose

I lose	Grams

After Waking up

Write your weight after wakeup

My Weight is	

In The Gym

Write the hours you spent in the gym

Gym Hours	

Before Sleeping

Write your weight before go to bed

My Weight is	

Lose weight

Subtract the 2 weights to know
how many grams you lose

I lose		Grams

After Waking up

Write your weight after wakeup

My Weight is	

In The Gym

Write the hours you spent in the gym

Gym Hours	

Before Sleeping

Write your weight before go to bed

My Weight is	

Lose weight

Subtract the 2 weights to know
how many grams you lose

I lose	Grams

After Waking up

Write your weight after wakeup

My Weight is	

In The Gym

Write the hours you spent in the gym

Gym Hours	

Before Sleeping

Write your weight before go to bed

My Weight is	

Lose weight

Subtract the 2 weights to know
how many grams you lose

I lose	Grams

After Waking up

Write your weight after wakeup

My Weight is	

In The Gym

Write the hours you spent in the gym

Gym Hours	

Before Sleeping

Write your weight before go to bed

My Weight is	

Lose weight

Subtract the 2 weights to know
how many grams you lose

I lose	Grams

After Waking up

Write your weight after wakeup

My Weight is	

In The Gym

Write the hours you spent in the gym

Gym Hours	

Before Sleeping

Write your weight before go to bed

My Weight is	

Lose weight

Subtract the 2 weights to know
how many grams you lose

I lose		Grams

After Waking up

Write your weight after wakeup

My Weight is	

In The Gym

Write the hours you spent in the gym

Gym Hours	

Before Sleeping

Write your weight before go to bed

My Weight is	

Lose weight

Subtract the 2 weights to know
how many grams you lose

I lose	Grams

After Waking up

Write your weight after wakeup

My Weight is	

In The Gym

Write the hours you spent in the gym

Gym Hours	

Before Sleeping

Write your weight before go to bed

My Weight is	

Lose weight

Subtract the 2 weights to know
how many grams you lose

I lose	Grams